PRETTY GIRL:

How To Be Really Pretty, Even If You Don't Think You Are

Bronwen Skye

Published by:

Cliostitch Publishing
P.O. Box 470604
Celebration, FL 34747

ISBN-10: 1533623929
ISBN-13: 9781533623928

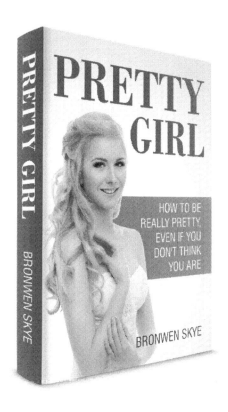

If you enjoy this book, and you would like to get the author's next book for free, simply visit http://bkrepublic.wix.com/pretty to sign up for a notification of publication. You can be one of the first to get it!! By signing up early, you'll get the Kindle version for free during the promotional launch!

DEDICATION

To my pretty sister

CONTENTS

INTRODUCTION

Warning: This book is about how to look outwardly pretty. In it I will be discussing things that you can do to maximize your beauty and gorgeousness. If you think that beauty is superficial and that looking pretty is unimportant or shallow, then this book is not for you.

I am not advocating beauty as a replacement for kindness or good behavior; in fact I am convinced that kindness and good behavior compliment a person's prettiness. I am also not saying that pretty is the be all and end all answer to life's trials, but I believe that it can surely help a girl in the world.

In this edition I will be talking a lot about how to maximize your outward appearance. If this offends you, put this book down and do not buy! For those of you who are ready to add pretty to your personal arsenal of life's ammunition, read on!!

1

WHY PRETTY?

WHAT DO YOU WANT?

Do you want guys to do a double take when you walk by? Do you want to be noticed when you walk into a room? Do you want women to be slightly envious because you're one of those pretty girls, and they wish they could be as pretty as you? If so, read on.

You may think that the only way a girl can be pretty is if she happens to win the genetic lottery. I am here to tell you that this just isn't the case. Oh, sure, there are a few women and girls who look pretty no matter what they do, but for the majority of us ladies there are ways around this. There are many movie stars and celebrities popular in media today who in reality just aren't that pretty, but it doesn't look like they're not beautiful; they just know how to work it.

I have also seen girls who have won those DNA sweepstakes, but you wouldn't know it to look at them. They look sloppy and disheveled. Their pretty is hidden. They may not even know that they have that golden ticket, and they may think that they are actually not pretty. You may be one of those girls. If so, you lucky lady, I will teach you to reveal your pretty.

I have also seen beautiful women who, if you look really closely you can tell that they didn't win that lottery. If you know what to look for, you can distinguish that really what you see is smarts and know-how. If you really don't feel like you have won that hereditary raffle, it's okay – the good news is, you can still be pretty! That's what I'm here to teach you.

Also, if you are not interested in reading my story, or you feel you have already mastered some of the sections in this book, then feel free to skip those segments and read on ahead to chapters that interest you.

MY STORY

My whole life, I've been fascinated by pretty girls. I saw that they were getting attention and perks that passed other girls by. There was also something unique and mysterious about them. I studied them for years and years, trying to figure out what made them different from other girls. I was trying to discover why they were the ones who were always in demand, being chased by a gaggle of men, while other girls sat on the sidelines with hardly a glance.

I did notice that there was a basic particular look – an ideal – that seemed to qualify as pretty (and I will tell you what that is in case you want to try it), but I also noticed that there were lots of girls who looked different from this ideal, who were still quite stunning, and who still seemed to get attention from men and envious glances from women. I studied them carefully to see what they had in common with the ideal that everyone seemed to think was so appealing.

I didn't start out thinking of myself as particularly pretty, but I desperately wanted to be. When I was young, people used to comment on my Shirley Temple curls and they wanted to pat my blonde head. They called me pretty, and I really liked this attention. They stopped doing this though, as I got older, and I missed it.

As a teenager I felt fairly powerless in the face of all the adults who were running my life. I felt like I had a controlling, domineering mother, and an angry father who didn't spend nearly enough time with me. I wanted power over something. I wanted power over the way people reacted to me. I saw that pretty girls had this. I saw that there were some girls like pale blonde Tammy who got everything she wanted just because she was conventionally pretty. She was really mean so I didn't like her, but she knew how to put herself together, which accentuated her pretty. I wasn't as pretty as she was at the time, because I didn't know her tricks. But older me knows I could have been if I'd known what I know now.

I also remember Marcella, who I badly wanted to be. Marcella was short, ethnic, and not very thin at all, but she was super nice and super popular and also extremely pretty. She knew how to put herself together. She knew all the tricks I'm about to tell you, and she used them. If you looked at photos of the two girls side by side, you might possibly think that Tammy was prettier than Marcella. But in real life Marcella was actually prettier than Tammy. But why? I was determined to find out.

Aside from wanting to be popular like the pretty girls, I also craved attention from men. I watched the movies and I observed the popular girls, and I knew that if you were pretty, you could get all the attention from men that you craved. I was determined to be one of those girls. I was constantly poring through books of pretty film stars. I would watch these stars again and again in movies, replaying the scenes where they really struck me as pretty, and trying to discern what it was that was making them that way.

When I moved to southern California in my twenties, I picked up a lot more info about pretty. They really know how to do it there. I remember the time I was dating a guy from another state. When he came to visit me in Cali, he looked around in awe at all the beautiful women. He said to me, "Wow, even the girls who aren't pretty are pretty here!" He was truly impressed. Bingo. It was true.

As I traveled to other states, I noticed more and

more that he was right. Many of the girls in other states just weren't as pretty as the girls in southern California. But it wasn't that they weren't born with any raw materials; it was just that they weren't using the tricks I was using. The things that had become second nature to me living in southern Cali, these girls didn't know how to use, or they didn't understand them. I always feel prettier in other states because I know the tricks that others do not, but I sure do like to look at the southern Cali girls and pick up more tricks for pretty.

SO WHAT DOES PRETTY GET YOU?

Once I started picking up the tricks in high school, my life became more like the fairy tale I imagined it could be. I definitely started enjoying more popularity, which thrilled me no end. I became one of those in-demand girls I'd always dreamed about.

I noticed I was getting tons of attention. The closer I came to cracking that pretty code, the more attention I got, and the more in-demand I was.

Girls were calling me on the phone to talk for hours (as we used to do in the pre-texting days), and boys were wanting to kiss me (and wanting to do other things as well). I didn't want to do all the other things that the boys wanted me to do, but I was very happy to have the option and the choice. I did start kissing a few boys though, with my new found popularity, and that was really fun too.

When I was in junior high, before I discovered the secrets of how to be pretty, I really wanted to be an actress. I was in drama class, and the drama teacher hardly noticed me. She barely gave me a two word line to read in class, and that was only because she was trying to include everyone. Not being noticed was super frustrating. How was I supposed to practice my craft, when I couldn't even get more than a line?

One time in drama class I remember being introduced to Christy, who was the lead in the high school play. I was so jealous; I really wanted to be her too. We had 5,000 kids in our school. As an invisible plain girl, I really had no hope of ever being cast in a play, much less as the lead. When I discovered how to be pretty, I got cast in every single play, and three times as the lead!

Life definitely got more interesting, and I hadn't had any plastic surgery or been abducted by aliens and sent back as Cindy Crawford – I'd just figured out how to fool people into thinking I was pretty, which is the same thing as being pretty. I already had the benefit of being thin, but I grew up vegetarian, so I knew I had a dietary advantage. Being veg is a great way to stay thin, which is usually the ideal. You can still be pretty if you're not thin, but thin just makes it easier.

Once I remember overhearing my younger sister talk about me in school. We were always butting heads at that age. She was exasperated with me, and said to someone in frustration, not understanding why I was getting all this attention, "She's not as pretty as everyone thinks she is!" And rather than the slap in the face this may have been meant to be, I took heart because I knew I was onto something. Not only could you use tricks to make yourself more attractive, but you could also fool people into thinking you were even prettier than you were.

Pretty girls do get the extra attention. They get the breaks in school. The teacher will stay after class or offer extra credit to someone who needs it if they are pretty. They should do it for everyone, and I am sure they try, but I sure got a lot more attention from my teachers when I was pretty than when I wasn't. It's easier to get attention if you're not invisible.

Pretty girls get other breaks too. Pretty girls can be really dumb and ask stupid questions, in school or real life, and people will stop and try to coach them. They will get a break instead of an eye roll. Why? Because everyone wants to be the one who's valuable to someone pretty. If pretty people pay attention to you, you feel special. I learned this whenever I felt the warm glow of Marcella's attention on me. I would have done anything for her. And yes, sometimes people will even do homework for pretty girls. I'm not saying it's ethical to let them!

Sometimes pretty girls get free stuff. Again, people just want to help pretty people; they want to be in their good graces. I don't know why – maybe it's an evolutionary thing – but I do know that it's true. As a pretty girl, I have had people give me all kinds of stuff for free: money, shoes, clothing, jewelry, services. In New York City I once had a cab driver waive the fare, just because I was pretty. That one really threw me, but it felt amazing.

I even had a sugar daddy once because I wanted to try it. Allow me to explain. In college I knew this beautiful black girl with long wavy hair who had a sugar daddy. She was always showing up with new jewelry, shoes, and clothes. The man was just a regular not-too-handsome white guy with money. I asked her if she had to sleep with him to get all this stuff. She said no, and I wasn't sure if I believed her. But she sure was pretty.

Fast forward a few years later and I had a sugar daddy of my own! It was crazy. He was taking me on trips with him, out to fancy dinners; he was buying me shoes, clothing, jewelry, and he even furnished my apartment. He was sending me large monthly checks. He was also one of those not-too-handsome white guys with money, just like my friend had.

And no, I actually did not have to sleep with him. He just wanted some arm candy and companionship. I was honestly shocked about that, but there it was. He kept saying he wished he had a daughter that he could spoil. I had to spend a lot of time with him whenever he came into town, but he never touched me sexually, it was never more than a peck on the cheek. He said he'd only do it if I wanted him to, and he was nice enough, but I really didn't like him that way.

I only kept up the sugar daddy thing for a few months. When I found out he had possible mafia connections, I got scared and ran. It wasn't too hard for me to extricate myself because I'd only given him a UPS Store address to send me the checks and a partial name, so he wasn't sure where I lived. I was blonde, but not dumb.

The point is, there are lots of things that pretty girls can get that are just not available to plain girls, and you can have them too. Are you ready to be a pretty girl?

2

GROOMING

THE BASICS

To be pretty, you definitely have to be well-groomed. Pretty girls always find the time to keep up with good grooming. This may seem obvious to some of you, but I've seen my share of otherwise attractive girls who look like they've literally just rolled out of bed. I understand the reasoning. Some girls want to have that wild, unkempt look. But to pull that look off, it actually takes a lot of work. Just rolling out of bed doesn't do it; the pretty girls just make it look that way.

I agree with that "just rolled out of bed" philosophy to some extent. Pretty has to look effortless; otherwise it can look gaudy or affected. If it shows that you're trying too hard, pretty gets lost. So I understand the confusion. People think, 'Well, that pretty girl just rolled out of bed and threw on some jeans and a tee shirt. She doesn't even look like she's trying.' Then those emulating girls try to do the same thing, and it just doesn't come across that way. What they don't realize is that this effortlessness is a carefully contrived art.

First of all, a pretty girl (even if it doesn't look this way because of Spray Dirt or whatever funky product she's using), is always freshly showered. She's clean and she smells nice and fresh, so no perfume is necessary. Pretty girls do sometimes use perfume, but not too much. They want to make it seem like they tried to be natural and clean – not like they purposefully dumped a whole flower shop on themselves. See, that's trying too hard. So, if you wear perfume, just spray it once into the air and step into it, and then there's just a faint lovely smell about you that could be mistaken for your natural smell. And pretty girls just smell nice. Because you're just pretty, right? You don't have to try.

Obviously you should also brush and floss. I know people don't floss as much as they say they do, if ever, but it needs to be done. Flossing keeps your teeth super pretty and clean and keeps your breath fresh. A pretty girl always has fresh breath. Like for-real fresh breath; not manufactured with mints or gum. Of course if you have immaculate dental habits and you eat an onion sandwich, mints or gum are okay for a quick fix. I prefer to use some pure peppermint oil mixed with water in a tiny little mist bottle. It's more natural-tasting, kills germs, and doesn't give you that gamey, synthetic, fake fresh.

Also, if you really hate flossing, I recommend trying a water pick. It's a bit of a messy water learning curve at first, but the warm water feels nice on your gums, which seems to make it less of a chore.

Flossing or using your water pick will keep your teeth in great shape, and beautiful teeth are key to pretty. If your teeth are not healthy, go get them fixed and then vow to take care of them; it's the only mouth you have! If your teeth are perfectly healthy but not quite so straight, consider an Invisalign consultation (which is covered by some insurances) or a consultation for porcelain veneers (which usually aren't). Either way, it's a wise investment. Straight, healthy teeth increase pretty exponentially.

NAILS

Nails ideally should be natural. If you really love fake nails and feel like your own aren't up to snuff, then go ahead and wear them. But don't be gaudy. Wear your nails no more than one quarter inch beyond your fingertips. Claw nails scare guys – and some girls too. There are guys out there that are actually completely grossed out by these long crazy fingernails. Do you remember the picture of the guy with the world's longest fingernails in *The Guinness Book of World Records*? That's what they think of. Ewww.

Pretty girls don't go much to extremes with their nails, like with nail art or stickers; they want it to look like they have more important things to do. And, of course they do, because since they are pretty, they are usually more popular. Pretty is more than just the outside, after all, but it helps if the outside is pretty too. That's what we're working on. So, the prettiest shape for nails is rounded square, not too round and not too square, just kind of in-between. Square with the edges rounded off, if you can wrap your nails around that.

Got it? Ok, moving on.

If you like to wear polish and you're under thirty, feel free to experiment with colors, but keep those nails short, especially if you choose some crazy hue. Otherwise stick to light reds, pinks, nudes, or go French. Older girls look prettier and younger in neutral tones.

Here's the thing about polish though: if it won't stay on your fingers, don't wear it! The second it starts chipping, get it re-done or take it off. Naked nails are way more the Tao for pretty girls than chipped polish, which always looks untidy and déclassé. Don't worry if your natural nails aren't perfect, just keep them short and clean and they'll look fine.

If you have trouble growing them at all, there's a great vitamin product out there called Skin, Hair, and Nails. It really works. It makes your nails tough and strong, increases the tensile strength of your hair, and helps your skin look nice. I know it works because when I take it my nails get so long they become a royal pain. I always have to file them down, and often. But I prefer that to the splitting, breaking nails I have when I don't take the supplement.

Toenails. Always groom your toenails. Unless your toenails grow super-fast, you probably only have to attend to them every 3-4 weeks. The great thing about toenails is that they are so super tough, that the polish usually stays on, yay! So make sure they are cut nice and short, but don't go too short and hurt yourself. And always, always, always have polish on them. They're your toes so you can use whatever colors you fancy. Most pretty girls tend to stick to reds, pinks or neutrals, but if you want something flashy, it's okay, as long as it doesn't start to chip. When it starts to chip, you need to get it off or re-touch.

Another style that pretty girls wear on their toes is a French manicure. This is always super classy and super cute. You really can't go wrong with it. You can do it in white or metallic, and it can look really sharp. Pretty girls always look properly manicured.

BODY HAIR

Okay pretty girls always shave their legs. At the very least they shave any part of their leg that is showing, so unless you always wear pants, below the knee is mandatory. I was once sitting next to a co-worker who works with a lot of women. He was a nice looking guy. I was wearing a dress and he actually thanked me for shaving my legs. I was kind of floored.

I must've looked really surprised because he felt the need to explain. "I'm serious," he said. "A lot of girls wear dresses or shorts and they don't even bother. I just really appreciate it. It looks like you care." So there you have it; pretty girls do care. They care about themselves of course, but they want to help others have a pleasant experience looking at them as well. What's the expression? Easy on the eyes.

Pretty girls shave their bikini lines regularly as well. If you never step into a bathing suit and you never see any action you can skip this step, unless it makes you feel unpretty. If it does, you should still keep the lawn looking trim. You don't have to go crazy with a

Brazilian wax unless that's what you want, but just shave the sides where errant hairs might be exposed under a bathing suit. The leaner design of the grassland makes you look slimmer in the nude as well.

If you have any dark facial hair you have to bleach it. Dark facial hair does not look pretty. Some girls even have dark hair that looks like sideburns – this needs to be bleached as well, or waxed. Everyone has some hair on their face, but if you don't like to have any hair at all above your lip, even if it's blonde, you can try epilating. Epilators pull the hair out by the roots so it grows back finer and sometimes not at all. Epilators can sting though when you use them, and if you have a sensitive face they can break you out at first, so test it on a small spot before you go full forward with that.

Many pretty girls have no hair above the lip, but I've been assured by the opposite sex that it is okay for girls to have a little bit of hair there if it is light or bleached. Also, if it's really thick, a pretty girl would try to get rid of it.

Make sure you don't have any errant nose hairs. Seriously, check. That's not pretty for guys or girls, especially if the hairs are dark. You can get a little precision eyebrow hair remover or a Finishing Touch shaver with a little light for about ten bucks. It is easy to get all those hairs with a tool like that without any pain whatsoever. If you want to pull them, it hurts like the dickens, but it's also effective.

If you have something crazy like back hair or really dark arm hair, you might want to look into professional waxing. I know that waxing and shaving isn't natural, but I'm just giving you the tools to be pretty in the twenty-first century. There's a basic idea about what constitutes pretty, and shaving is included.

You can also consider electrolysis or laser hair removal for any parts of your body hair that are troubling you if you don't want to shave every day and you don't like epilators or waxing. Sometimes these options can be expensive, but it sounds really nice to never have to worry about it again.

EYEBROWS

Also make sure your eyebrows aren't too crazy. The brows frame your beautiful eyes like a fine piece of art. You cannot have a unibrow and be a pretty girl. Look carefully at your brows in the mirror and pluck all the ones that are off by themselves or clearly don't belong. Mostly just pluck below the brow. Try to avoid plucking above it unless you have a really crazy hair or two up there. Brows look best when they are higher on the face. Having them too close to your peepers will make your eyes look small and not give them the proper frame they deserve.

If you want to go for a natural look, that can be pretty. But remember: natural; not wild. If they are thick that's okay, but they have to be controlled. If they are really wily, make sure you use some brow gel to tame them. On the other hand, if you prefer a more architectural look, and you don't want to go to a professional (which is definitely something that would be recommended), there are brow guides out there that you can buy to help you tweeze a good shape. Just try to stick to the rules, and tweeze under you brows; not over.

By the same token you don't want brows that are too tiny and thin, so don't over-pluck. That style is so nineteen thirties and looks really dated today. Also, be warned that sometimes those hairs never grow back. You just want a nice middle-of-the-road thickness (unless you're Brooke Shields). If you want to go thinner it's okay, just make sure they're bigger than a toothpick. Most of all, you want your brows to look clean and groomed just like the rest of you. Good grooming is the hallmark of pretty girls everywhere, even when they try to pretend like they just rolled out of bed.

3

HAIR

COLOR

Hair color is a passionate topic that has a lot to do with a woman's identity. Women identify with their hair color, and they are most often identified by it. They say, "I'm a redhead," or, "My friend is a brunette," and, "That woman is a blonde." So hair colors don't describe what you have so much as what you are. This is interesting because of course your hair color has nothing to do with who you are on the inside. Or does it?

I've spent some time living in different hair colors. Namely, blonde, brunette, red, and black. Once for a few days I even had purple hair, but that's another story. Pretty girls tend to stick to the basic colors. If you actually are Katy Perry, you can wear blue hair, but remember that she started out as a very pretty brunette, and we learned to think of her as pretty before she changed her color so dramatically. Once you are established as a bona fide pretty girl, you have more license to do as you please and still be identified in that special group. In any case, I can sincerely tell you that I felt different in every single one of those colors. Not only did I feel different, but I was treated differently.

I have been light golden blonde most of my life. I can honestly say that I feel the best and most like myself when I'm blonde. I feel like I have a halo of light around my face. As a blonde in my younger days women tended not to trust me as much, but the attention from men, the first time I went blonde, was off the charts. Blonde, all by itself, is a head turner. I believe that women didn't trust me as much because as an unattached younger blonde they perceived me as pretty (whether I was or not) and subconsciously felt like I was going to try and steal their boyfriends!

As a chocolatey brunette I wasn't as noticeable to men, they kind of looked past me, and I didn't get as many offers for dates and such coming at me like gang busters. The guys I did attract though were of respectable quality. Quality over quantity – brunette vs. blonde, good to know. Women tended to trust me more and revealed more of their secrets to me, much to my surprise. I believe this is because they were no longer threatened by me.

As a fiery redhead I was mostly trusted by both men and women, and the guys did seem to dig it. I got a lot of compliments – more from men than women, but women were cool with it too. And guys who were into red were very into red.

People's reaction to the black hair was kind of a combo between being a brunette and a redhead. I got more attention from men than as a chocolate brunette, but not as much as when I was a redhead. Women trusted me, but not quite as much as when I was chocolate. I also felt very edgy and goth. There's a cool vibe to having raven black hair, and I attracted edgier guys.

The truth is you can be pretty with any of the basic hair colors. However, the quintessential pretty girl has always been blonde, so I consider this a cheat or shortcut. Most of the fairy tales in olden days began with a flaxen maiden of some kind. Admittedly, Disney's first princess was a brunette, but if Snow

White could have been blonde, I'm sure she would have been. There was a clear predilection for blondes at the company's outset with Sleeping Beauty, Cinderella, and even Tinkerbell. Then, as if sensing they needed some serious princess diversity, Disney started to more regularly introduce royalty with other hair colors.

If you really feel like you identify better with colors other than blonde and you don't want to cheat with a hair color, that's fine; you can still be pretty with other tricks. But you might consider getting some blonde highlights just to give yourself a hint of that magic potion. Maybe even just a tiny bit in the front. I'm telling you, it works. However, don't do this if you have really dark hair and plan to keep it. If your hair is black or super dark brown, you should work that dark and mysterious beauty angle. Blonde will only mess it up.

CUT

If your hair is reasonably healthy, don't cut it, except for trims. Guys love long hair, and women envy it. Long hair is another one of those cheats. Long hair is immediately identified with beauty, no matter what the color. If you have long, healthy hair you are immediately ahead of the game and should consider yourself lucky.

If you don't have long hair, try to grow it. If you can't grow long hair, consider getting some hair extensions. They can help you be wicked pretty. And yes, you can get the really expensive semi-permanent kind that they have in salons, glued, sewn, or braided in, or you can just use the less expensive clip in or flip in extensions.

Be careful though: they have to match your hair color precisely in order for it to look realistic. Believe me, people will notice you if you wear them. If you pull this off and match extensions correctly, you will literally feel people looking at you and lusting after your beautiful hair.

If you are African American and you don't like your natural hair, you ladies have a free license to use extensions and even wigs that Caucasian girls just don't have. By all means get an awesome gorgeous weave. You don't have to worry about it looking fake in the same way that Caucasians do; somehow it just works on you. With weaved-in hair, you don't really even have to worry about which color it is (by all means go blonde if you want to), because of the sheer volume of long hair, you're going to look gorgeous.

If you have alopecia, or you heave another medical condition that prevents you from having any hair at all, invest in a killer wig. You are going to have to spend a little money to get it to look real enough, but companies like Jon Renau have some surprisingly affordable lace top wigs, which is what you would want.

All one length of hair is the most versatile, and is very conventionally pretty, so I always recommend that. But if you have really thick hair then some long layers should also look beautiful on you. If you really like to rock the short do, just know it's not a quick fix to pretty. You have to be bold and confident to pull this off. You can still be pretty, but you'll have to rely on other tricks. Maybe try a platinum blonde.

If you have a high forehead, or even a really short

one, you might consider getting some bangs. They can help disguise the parts of your brow that don't seem as pretty as the rest of your face. Also, if you are an older girl and feel like there are some wrinkles getting in your way of pretty, grown-up stars like Goldie Hawn and Christie Brinkley prove that pretty can have bangs. But please have them cut by a professional and don't go too short. Bang disasters can send pretty to the hospital for a few weeks to take her sweet time to recover.

HAIRSTYLE

This is the hair necessity that trumps all others. You have to style your hair. Good style is crucial to pretty. If you have long blonde hair and it looks crazy and fried, you are not going to look as pretty as a well-coiffed short haired brunette. But even if your hair really is fried, fortunately there are some things you can do to make it look lovely.

First of all, if your hair is oily at the roots even a couple of hours after you shower, make sure you are using a dry shampoo, like Batiste. This sprays powder at the roots which absorbs all the oil for a reasonably long time. Pretty girls have clean looking roots. Take care to fluff your hair really well where you sprayed, and rub your fingers through your roots to distribute the powder evenly. You don't want to look as if you have dandruff.

Also, if you are a really pale blonde, talcum powder will work for this as well. If you are light blonde and your roots keep getting brassy, talcum powder will also take that brass out and make them look white again. If you use talc though you are going to need a shine spray so the rest of your hair does not look dull.

Next, if your hair is naturally curly and you like to wear it that way, I recommend the book Curly Girl by Lorraine Massey for in-depth care and styling suggestions. Otherwise, your hair will look beautiful if you use a straightening tool like the Instyler, or a waving iron like the Kiss Insta-Wave. Both products are killer.

If you feel like your hair always looks crappy no matter what you do, I have a cheat for that: hair pieces.

Before you start thinking about William Shatner, let me tell you that they have come a long way in recent years and some of them have the benefit of looking incredibly realistic. They help you look like you have a crazy gorgeous head of hair without wearing a full wig. Can you say modern princess?

It is super important though that you have an undetectable match. The only way to do this for sure is to order a color ring. Many wig companies like Vogue Wigs have a loaner program where you can pay the $30 for the ring and then send it back for a $30 credit once you pick out your perfect color. I prefer to keep my color rings though, in case my color changes slightly so I can keep getting a match.

I have tried Luxhair, Revlon, Tony of Beverly, Hairdo, HairUWear, Put On Pieces, Raquel Welch, Forever Young, Paula Young, Dancing with the Stars, and probably a few others. The most realistic synthetic pieces I have found by far are from a company called Easihair. Their colors are truly complimentary to most, and their pieces are convincing. You can look like you have a gorgeous movie star ponytail in 5 minutes flat, with no curling or ironing. Just buy the ring, match the color, and choose. When you get your piece in, you will look stunning with almost no effort.

The pieces I am talking to you about now are synthetic. They have a couple of advantages over human hair. One, they are much cheaper. Two, they always keep their style, rain, shine or humidity. Human hair, though thicker, will act like your own and respond to the weather. It's better if it doesn't. Synthetic pieces may look a little too shiny when you first get them, but you already have a bottle of dry shampoo on hand, right? Just mist them down with that and fluff.

As a side note, most of the pieces come with both jaw clip and fusion style. I find the jaw clips (though slightly easier to install) to be a little bulky looking. If you truly want that seamless convincing look, make sure you buy fusion pieces with the two little combs and a drawstring, and take that bulky clip out. It looks so much more realistic.

So let's say you have crappy frizzy hair and you don't want to – or don't feel like – wearing hair pieces or curling or straightening you hair. What can you do?

Here's where you have your secret weapon. You need to create one Go-to Updo. Try as many styles as many times as you like. When you hit one that flatters you, do it again and again and again until you get really good at it. Use it when you just can't make it look right another way. I've gotten so good at mine that people think it took me hours to create, when instead it only takes minutes – sometimes one minute if I'm lucky.

I've found some beautiful styles to copy and play around with in a book called "Vintage Hairstyles". I like vintage styles because they are timeless and outlive all the trends, so conversely you never look old fashioned. There are also YouTube videos galore on creating a fabulous updo. Like I said, you don't need to get good at all of them – just one – and you will always look classy and pretty.

4

MAKEUP

FOUNDATION

Now I'm going to talk to you about a part of every pretty girl's arsenal: makeup. And here's the truth about makeup: it's there to enhance what you have; it's not there to make you look like an overdone harlot. The idea is that you want to look naturally pretty, and as though you have hardly any makeup on at all. But the reality is that in order to look pretty by modern standards, everyone needs a little something.

I know that some girls get really excited about makeup, and other girls balk at the very idea of putting anything on their face. If you're in the first group, this will be easy for you; your main challenge will be to avoid overdoing it. For those of you in the second group, my challenge is going to be to convince you to put on just a little bit. So, let's start with the basics, let's talk about foundation.

Less is more. Some of you have perfect skin and can get away with no foundation at all, but most of us need a little help in that area. Of course, you don't want it to look like you have on any foundation. You want it to look like you just naturally have perfect skin, and if you already have perfect skin then congratulations, you might be able to skip this step with just a little bit of tweaking. You definitely don't want it to look like you're wearing foundation, so I always recommend lighter versions of foundations like BB creams and tinted moisturizers. Some of these even have sunscreens in them, which can be really helpful in keeping your face looking fresh and pretty.

For color, always go with lighter shades if you're in-between two choices. BB creams and tinted moisturizers usually only come in a few highly-compatible shades, so it shouldn't be too difficult to narrow it down. Don't go with the darker one unless you're going to use it as a contour, and even then you have to be careful. Dark foundation will show up like tribal face paint. On the other hand, you don't want to look like a ghost either. Choose carefully.

You want the color to be as close to your skin color as is humanly possible to make it look like that perfect canvas is actually your skin. You may have to try a few of the tinted moisturizers and BB creams to hit on one that really works for you. A plain moisturizer is okay to use as well if the colors just aren't cutting it for you.

Once you find one, this is the step to begin with. Blend it into your face, but not your eyelids, before applying other makeup. You want your eye makeup to stick and not slide off. If you have really great looking skin, you can skip this step. We will get into the tweaking later on. Once you have on that foundation, moisturizer or BB cream that makes your skin look really lovely, you can start getting down to the artistry.

BROWS

I read a book by Raquel Welch which suggested that after foundation, you should always start with your brows. I never used to do that, and I thought it was silly at the time, but now I always start with my brows. Brows frame the face and are more important than most people give them credit for. It would really be better to go without eyeshadow than to go without brow powder or at least brow gel. It's really essential that they look natural. You don't want any of that cartoonishly penciled-in ridiculousness.

I'd like to stress again you don't want it to look like you're wearing makeup. What you want is to look like you're really pretty without it, as we discussed in the earlier chapter. You also don't want it to look like your brows are out of control. So grab an appropriately colored gel or a pencil, and with light feathery strokes carefully fill in any place in your natural brow that you're missing. I recommend E.L.F.'s brow kits – they are inexpensive and work like a charm.

Once you've done that, you can take a brow powder (included in the E.L.F. kits) that's a bit lighter than your brows but close to your natural color (again, you never want to go too dark), and carefully sweep a little bit of that all over your brows in the same manner. Always try to follow the natural line of your brow, and don't try to make your brows into something that they are not. Just make them look full and healthy, because that's pretty. Also, if your brows tend to get a little unruly, make sure you put some clear brow gel on top of your brow arch to hold them in place – at least gel the parts that get crazy.

EYESHADOW

Now for your eyeshadow. It's imperative that you have natural looking eyes. You can sometimes wear crazy colors, especially if you're under thirty, but you have to be careful about doing this. You don't want to look like a clown; clowns aren't pretty. If you're going to use any colors other than nudes, browns, or taupes (which I highly recommend), make sure that you never ever put them above your crease. If you're going to wear crazy colors, they belong on the lid only or as a liner.

Some cosmetic companies have come out with lining potions that can turn any eyeshadow into a liner, or you can just use water to mix; this works especially well with baked eyeshadows. So if you have that crazy teal color that you've been dying to try, only put a little bit of it on the outer third of your eye, as liner, or over your entire lid if you really want to go wild. The pretty girls will usually use it as an eyeliner.

Before you get started with your eyes, always use a shadow primer first on your eyelid to keep your eyeshadow looking fresh. Then line your upper eyelashes. Take a black or dark brown (preferably creamy) pencil, and blend it as near to your lashes as you can get. Try to get as close to in between the lashes as you can with it on top of your eyelid to make your lashes look really full. Then it's best to blur it slightly, ombré style, with a smudge brush.

There are a couple of ways pretty girls do their eyeshadow. This first look is a natural look eyeshadow that deepens and accentuates your eyes. For this technique you can use two or three neutral colors. Take a light nude color and brush it all over your lid and brow. Now just accent with a slightly darker color in the darkest part of your crease. Blend well. Always blend, blend, blend. Then if you want to use a third color, take the darkest color and, with a small slanted brush, use it as an eyeliner, setting the cream eyeliner you used before you applied the powder.

This next technique works if you want to create a smoky eye. You will need three colors for this one. Again, apply a light nude color all over your lid and brow. Then, choose a medium color to apply all over your lid, and a little bit up into the outer crease. Then take your darkest color and apply it over your original cream eyeliner to create depth and dimension. You can even blend a little bit of the dark shadow into the outer third corner of your lid and crease. Voilà, smoky eyes. I recommend you mainly stick with brownish smoky eyes if you are over thirty, while under thirty girls can also successfully use a white, black, and gray palette.

You have probably been told this before, but it bears repeating: always make a choice. If you are going with any dark makeup at all, go with dark eyes and light lips, or light eyes and dark lips. Never ever go with dark lips and dark eyes; you will look way too overdone, and like you are trying too hard. Pretty needs to look effortless. If you want to go for the red lips, that's fantastic – just make sure you have a natural, toned-down eye. Marilyn Monroe was famous for her red lips, but she always wore a neutral, natural eye with a bit of liner. If you want to have an incredibly sultry smoky eye that's fine, but make sure you have a really natural light lip.

Also, red glosses and tinted lipsticks are easier to wear than flat out red lipstick. If you are under thirty and you can really rock the matte red, go for it. Older girls need to be careful not to go too dark because this can make them look older or harsher. If you are older, always try to bring light to your face to flatter it, and this includes your lips.

THE REST

After you finish your eyeshadow, this is the perfect time for face tweaking. First, take a fan brush and brush away any stray powder from the eyeshadow that may have fallen under your eyes or onto your cheeks. Then take a little bit of light colored foundation or BB cream and apply it under your eyes. Place a little arc of foundation under your eyes and blend to get rid of any trace of circles or puffiness. Then you might want to put a little bit of foundation between your eyes or in the folds of your nose or anywhere else that might be a little bit reddish. Blend well. If you have any blemishes to cover up that your BB cream didn't quite get, this is the time to do it.

I don't recommend using foundation face powders at all because they just make you look like an old lady, and it looks really makeup-y. Again, you don't want to look like you're wearing makeup. Now if you're into contouring, this is the time to do it. You can put a little contour under your cheekbones, in the crease of your eye, along the sides of your nose, or anywhere else that you would like recessed.

Cream blush looks more natural than powder, so put a little splash of cream blush on the apples of your cheeks or along cheekbones and blend well. This could be really light; it doesn't have to be anything heavy, just a tiny splash of peach or pink. Don't blend it all the way to your hairline; that looks really obvious and amateurish.

Now is the time to use your powder highlighter.

Powder highlighter's purpose is twofold: one is to set the makeup you've already used, and two is to give your face that three dimensional look. Places to use your highlighter are on your brow bone, along the bridge of your nose, on your cheekbones, and right above your upper lip. Maybe a little bit on your forehead if it looks right on you.

Obviously with all these makeup tips, you need to keep in mind that you want to accentuate the positive. So, if you have wonderful gorgeous eyes, please accentuates those. If you have amazing lips, do not pay as much attention to the eyes and definitely focus on those lips. If you have high cheekbones highlight those, and if you have beautiful brows make those the stars.

Lastly, of course make sure you use mascara. Mascara opens your eyes and makes you look awake. Many girls can't really get away with using mascara or liner on their bottom lashes, so some pretty girls just skip this all together. You don't want the black to come bleeding down later so that you end up looking like Frankfurter from the Rocky Horror Picture Show. On that note, make sure you choose a mascara that is not going to run.

My favorite mascara is Kiss Me Mascara by Blink. This stuff very rarely comes off until you take it off. If it ever does come off, it's just in tiny flakes. It doesn't ever run – it can't – that's not the way it's built. To remove, just rub it off gently with warm water and light pressure and the little tubes just fall right off your lashes. If you use this mascara you will never ever get raccoon eyes unless you use a bottom liner, which I don't recommend. If a bottom liner bleeds your dark circles will just look ridiculous, and not pretty at all. If you feel you must use a liner on the bottom anyway, I recommend using a lighter color like pink or bronze that won't create raccoon eyes.

Also, if you feel like wearing false eyelashes, put them on after the mascara, and make sure you only use them on the outer half or third of the eye, otherwise they may look fake. Just cut them to fit and glue. It may take some practice.

With the idea that you're just naturally pretty and you don't want makeup to look like makeup, try to follow this tenant: Just use a splash of color. Don't go loco with all the crazy new colors and the trends of the season; that's just used to sell magazines to women who don't know how to be pretty.

What you want is something to make you look like you're naturally pretty, and to bring out your own natural beauty. A light hand is best and is always better than a heavy one, and so when in doubt use less.

5

SKINCARE

BASIC SKINCARE

Part of being really pretty is having the best skin you can possibly have for you. Does it have to be flawless for you to be pretty? Thank goodness it doesn't. But we'd like to make it as close to flawless as possible to stack the pretty odds in our favor.

You've probably been told all of your life to wash off your make-up before going to bed. If you are a bona fide pretty girl using these techniques, you are probably going to be wearing make-up. Why is washing your face at the end of the day so important? Well, it's essential to wash off not only your make-up, which can be tiring and stressful to skin, but also any environmental stressors of the day.

We are talking about smoke, fumes, volatile organic compounds, and free radicals. These things are hard on skin, and your skin likes to take a rest and do what it does best: repair itself! It really wants to and is programmed to do this, we just need to help it along.

You've probably also heard that you should never wash your face with regular soap. For years I ignored this tenet. This was to my detriment. I had skin problems for years and was determined to scrub off the bacteria as roughly and thoroughly as I could. Little did I know that I was upsetting my already delicate skin even more, and making it nearly impossible for it to do its job by stripping it of the protections it kept trying to build for me every night.

Use a gentle cleanser to wash off your make-up. Coconut oil works well for eye make-up remover. Some people can even use it all over their face to cleanse their skin. It is too oily for me as a cleanser, but you will have to try out different cleansers for yourself to determine what's right for you. Find one that you can use that doesn't irritate your skin, maybe even one that is gentle on your eyes. If it doesn't hurt your eyes, it won't harm your skin.

Back in the day, common wisdom indicated that we should wash our faces twice a day. Now dermatologists are suggesting that we really shouldn't do much to our faces in the morning by way of cleansing. Some skin docs now say that the best thing to do in the morning is to wash your skin with water only and then air dry, or gently pat dry. Again, there is a protective barrier that your skin has worked hard to build up during the night to protect your face and keep it supple looking. Don't rain on its parade; it's trying to help you!

In the morning you can use your moisturizer if you need it. Hopefully you have found a light one that works for you. If a heavy one works for you, by all means, use that. It is also a good idea to wear some sort of protection or sunscreen during the day to keep your skin looking its best. You can use a commercial sunscreen if that is what you feel comfortable doing. I would also like to point out that some cultures use coconut oil or sesame oil as a natural sunscreen. This has the added benefit of moisture for the skin, a protective barrier to environmental stresses, and it is irritant free.

Personally, I like to use the natural oils most of the time. I use virgin coconut oil mixed with a few drops of essential oils. If I am going to spend a day in the sun where my face is really exposed, I will always opt for a commercial sunscreen made specifically for faces. Coconut oil is not strong enough keep your face free from burns on a sunny beach day!

At night it is also a good idea to help your skin stay nourished with a moisturizer of some kind. Again, if I feel I need it, I like to use the coconut oil as a light protective barrier after I cleanse my face. Some girls may not even need to use very much – just a smidge.

If your skin is really dry or in need of exfoliation, do it, but do it gently. Exfoliation should only be done once or twice a week at most. When you do this you remove the skin's protective barrier and it has to grow new skin. This can occasionally be beneficial, but constant scrubbing can just make it irritated, recalcitrant and cranky. You want to treat your skin gently and keep it happy.

SKIN EMERGENCIES

Sometimes, despite your best efforts and kindly

overtures to your skin, your skin rebels and you have what I like to refer to as a skin emergency. Your skin breaks out in tiny red dots, you get a rough red patch, or worse – a volcano brewing deep within its center. There are several ways to deal with these and I will go over them.

The number one tenet of dealing with skin emergencies is do not pick! I know the temptation is incredible to do so. You just want it to go away and you want to make it right so you feel if you squeeze or pick the living daylights out of it, it will go away. But the skin requires patience and a gentle hand or it can turn around and royally screw you.

This is what happens when you pick: Your skin is already upset and doesn't like that, so it turns red first of all. If your friends and family might not have noticed that spot on the side of your face, they surely will now because it is bright red from irritation, it will show up a lot worse, and be more difficult to cover.

Then, sometimes in trying to relieve the pressure of a blemish, we squeeze it. If we are lucky we may get some release of pressure on the outside, but likely if it is not clearly ready to blow, it will also get squeezed on the inside, pushing the infection into deeper layers of the skin and making it last much longer than if you had just left it alone.

Never try to get the yucky stuff out unless it is without a doubt, full on, ready to go. You are asking for trouble if you do otherwise. If you decide it is really ready, be sure to use an extractor tool and never your fingers.

Fortunately, there are several things you can do in the meantime. I have found that essential oils work best for me in these types of emergencies. If you are looking at something cystic, I recommend trying clove essential oil. It is really strong, and not all skin types can take it. My skin can only take a few applications, but clove is a drawing oil and will draw infection to the surface. Peppermint oil and tea tree oils also work to kill infections. If you have really sensitive skin you might try lavender oil. This oil is an all-around balm and healer of skin, and it is also anti-infectious.

A word about essential oils: they are not all created equal. Be careful what you put on your face.

Try to use food grade or therapeutic grade oils if you can find them. DoTerra Essential Oils are the ones I use most often and I trust them to be pure.

Other things you can apply to your skin are cortisone cream to bring down the swelling, and silver gel to help with rapid healing. Hopefully one of these things will work for you. I have had blemishes that responded to clove oil overnight, and some that have taken a week to get rid of. The nice thing about attacking them with essential oils though is that you know blemishes are there, but it is tough for others to see them because you are not making a crazy mess of them. When your face is not trashed from picking, the spots are relatively easy to cover up.

What else can you do if you are still going crazy from a skin emergency? There are some quick fixes for that too. Anti-inflammatories like Advil can temporarily bring down the swelling of your blemish. Also, if you really can't stand your blemishes, try taking antihistamines for a day or two. These really calm down the skin and get it back to fighting the good fight. As with all medication, even over the counter ones, know if they are right for you, follow the directions and use with care.

What if you have a nasty bump or skin tag on your face? Well, definitely get it removed by a dermatologist! However, there is a way you can get rid of them on your own, but you have to be very careful. I want to make it clear that I am not recommending that you do this, only making you aware of a product. This product called black salve. It is bloodroot mixed with zinc and it is very powerful stuff. I have removed several bumps from my face and body using this. If you are determined to use this stuff despite all government warnings, try it on another body part first before applying anything to your face.

Here is the way I have used it: One needs to rough up the spot with a sterile nail file, just a little so it breaks up the top layer of skin, no need to bleed. Then one applies the salve for two to five minutes only for the face. I have seen websites that suggest leaving it on for twenty-four hours and keeping it covered for weeks. This is not only unnecessary but harmful and can result in scarring. Do not keep it covered (unless you need to for going out), but keep applying moisture to it as often as possible. Neosporin works well for this. It will fall off and heal usually with one to three weeks, depending. It can possibly look rather nasty during weeks two though three, so plan accordingly.

It is also good to note when using this product that if it is working you will feel a slight stinging sensation. If you do not feel this while it is on your skin, it may not have worked and you may have to apply again at a later time. How do you know that it worked after you wash it off? The spot will darken or give some visible clue that effect has been taken. A pure brand is available from Best on Earth products. It is pricy but will last a very long time. Again, I'm not recommending this dangerous stuff to anyone, but it worked for me.

ANTI-AGING

What if you are not a teenager or twenty-something anymore and you have some wrinkles? Or what if you are wrinkling prematurely but don't really feel that injections and plastic surgery are right for you? There are things you can do to look younger and prettier without taking such drastic steps.

If you have read the chapter up to this point, you may already be using sunscreens and moisturizers on your face. This is a great place to start. Sunscreens of some kind are more important as you get older, since your skin doesn't repair itself with the same tenacity it did when you were younger.

Coconut oil is said to be an effective skin rejuvenator and wrinkle fighter. This is my moisturizer of choice. I like to add a few drops of Lavender and Frankincense essential oils to my coconut oil to help with anti-aging. The good news is that there are many essential oils that work really well for aging skin, and you can experiment to create your own special blend.

Retinol is a great skin regenerator and wrinkle fighter that you can use topically. It increases cell production in the top layer of skin, so skin looks younger because the cells are new, and you have increased turnover. Because skin uses retinoic acid when it produces collagen, it also provides a collagen boost. It is best to only use it once a day or only at night and ease yourself into it as it can be irritating at first. It is very important to use sunscreen if you are using this product in your beauty arsenal.

If your skin can take it, you can use topical magnesium to ease wrinkles. Be careful with this mineral salt because it can also irritate the skin and may not be for everyone. Magnesium relaxes muscles whereas Botox incapacitates them. I'd rather have my muscles relax. There are brands out there made with aloe vera to ease the sting.

Also there is a product called Smoothies. They are little pieces of non-adhesive tape that train your face to relax where you have wrinkles. You wear them at night, and wake up to a fresh canvas. Throughout the day your wrinkles will return, but if you use them often enough you can re-train your face to look more carefree.

Additionally, I would recommend taking an oral supplement. Skin, Hair and Nails, the same one you take for your nails, is also good for your skin. Vitamin

E supplements are also beneficial. Try different brands and find one that works for you to get that extra nourishment from the inside.

But here's the truth: nothing will refresh your skin more than a good night's sleep. So make sure you are getting your zzz's. There is a reason why they call it a beauty sleep. The body uses that time to rejuvenate itself in ways that we can only dream of when we are awake. So make sure you get a good night's slumber as often as possible. In other words, make sure you get your pretty rest.

6

DIET AND EXERCISE

DIET

In order to keep yourself as pretty as possible, you need to think about daily maintenance of that pretty form of yours. First, we're going to talk about what sorts of things pretty girls eat to keep themselves pretty. The optimal diet for a pretty girl is a preponderance of fruits and vegetables! Fruits and vegetables will not only keep you slim because they have hardly any calories, but they are nutritional power houses as well.

Will plants make you pretty? Yes!! Eat as many of them as you can! Researchers at the University of St. Andrews in Scotland did two studies showing that consuming vegetables significantly increased their subject's attractiveness factor by creating a rosy glow in skin color that ramped up their subject's desirability meter.

The University of Nottingham did a similar study and found that eating lots of fruits and vegetables caused the skin to have a natural glow. This glow was caused primarily by carotenoids in the veggies, and was visible after subjects ate seven or more servings of vegetables a day for as little as six weeks. A typical serving is about a cup of leafy greens or a half cup of other veggies.

Michael Pollan, in his book *In Defense of Food: An Eater's Manifesto*, says this: "Eat food. Not too much. Mostly plants." Plants are the foods humans are ideally suited to eat. They come straight from nature in the perfect nutritional amounts for us. If we eat mostly fruits and vegetables, we will be thin and also have all of the nutrition we need to keep our skin healthy and beautiful.

I'd like to point out that these foods are best taken in their whole entire forms. That means you eat the apple and the skin, the potato and the skin, the florets of the broccoli and the stalk. As much as is possible for you to eat of the entire plant, eat it. Nature has devised it so we get the perfect amounts of everything we need if we just eat the whole plant. If a part of the plant is too tough or too bitter to eat, it is probably a part of it that we are not supposed to eat anyway, like onion peels or avocado skins (which are mildly toxic).

If you just eat the inside of the potato or apple, you are missing out on all the great minerals in the skin of the plant. Just eating the skins would probably be yucky, and you'd be missing out on the carbs you need to keep your beautiful engine running. Eating the whole plant not only applies to fruits and vegetables, but it also applies to grains. We are talking about whole grain brown rice and whole grain brown wheat. If you look for products that include the entire plant, it's tough to go wrong. These products are infinitely less fattening than their white counterparts and have tons more nutrition.

Brown rice is easy to find. Whole grain wheat is a little tougher to find. You have to look for the words whole grain wheat, and not just whole wheat. If you are in a pinch though, whole wheat is better than white. I have found that *Food For Life Ezekiel* products are a perfect fit. They are sprouted whole grains, a complete protein by themselves and they contain everything you need including all nine essential amino acids to nourish you and keep you healthy. The sprouting also helps with digestion, and anything that helps with digestion will keep your tummy slim. If you have a gluten allergy, just look for whole grains that don't include wheat. *Food For Life* makes sprouted gluten free breads as well.

Let's talk about dairy for a second. This is a good place to remind you of what cow milk is originally intended for. Cow milk is intended to grow a sixty pound baby calf into a thousand plus pound cow in two to three years. That's literally half a ton! Some cows grow to be a full ton or more. This food is intended to put an enormous amount of weight on a large boned animal in a short amount of time. This is weight that pretty girls can do without.

Not to mention that Colin T. Campbell proves in his bestselling book, *The China Study*, that dairy causes heart disease, diabetes, and even cancer. Whole, skim, and nonfat varieties are all guilty of this. How awful is that? He could literally turn on and off cancer by feeding dairy to his subjects and then retracting the dairy. Seriously, cow dairy is not for any humans, and especially not for pretty girls. There are lots of great dairy alternatives out there – find one that works for you, and minimize this serious bulker upper.

Because you are so busy stuffing yourself with all the fruits and vegetables you can find, does this mean that you can't ever have that stray piece of chocolate cake? Of course not. If you are truly eating lots of fruits and vegetables you probably won't have too much room for stuff that's not healthy for you. But you shouldn't go on an absolute strike of the foods that you love. Allow yourself to have a little bit of them from time to time. Just a little bit when you really want it, like maybe some dark chocolate after dinner. If you go on a complete food strike, your pretty regimen won't last.

Here's the thing too: you can't think of it as a diet. Think of it as a way of life. Eat as many fruits and veggies as you can (and you cannot possibly eat too many so go ahead and chow!) and then if you want a little something else like cake or wine now and then, then go for it. If you make it your modus operandi, then you are never really on a diet; that's just how you eat. And unlike with a diet, you are never really restricting yourself too much to keep it up.

So what do pretty girls do when they go to a restaurant? You probably already know the answer. They order the salad. This is what you should do too. Order an entrée size salad, and eat it. Everyone else at the table will be envious. That's just the way it works. They will look at your beautiful salad and they will always say that they should have ordered it too. The more vegetables in your salad the more your companion diners will look at you with envy. They will look at you, pretty girl, and know one of the reasons you are so pretty.

Back in the day, all salads were mostly vegetables. Now that's not always the case, and sometimes it seems tough to find one with lots of veggies. If all the salads on the menu are animal protein centric, one thing you can do is go through the menu, especially the list of salads, and write down all the veggies they have that you would like to see in your salad. Hand the list to the waiter and ask nicely if they will make all this lovely stuff they already have into a special salad for you. I've never been refused.

What if you are still hungry? Then get something else. A side dish, perhaps some naughty french fries if you really want them. Maybe even a little dessert if you can't help yourself. But you were already good and you ate your salad, so now you can have a little of something else you want. Your veggie quota has already been met so you are good to go. You've already impressed everyone by ordering the salad, so no one will judge you if you eat a few french fries.

Here's another tip: one bite in the evening's worth two in the morning. And it only gets worse the later you go. What does this mean? Ideally, don't eat late. Everything you eat before five o'clock will be mostly burned off by bedtime. Everything you eat after five will stick to your hips and belly. So what can you do about that? You can eat a really good sized breakfast and/or lunch, and a light dinner. Remember that calories count less when you eat them before five. After five is when you pack on the pounds. So that chocolate cake would be better as a lunchtime treat than after dinner. Just keep this little secret in mind.

EXERCISE

Now let's talk about exercise. Do all pretty girls literally kill themselves at the gym to get those killer bodies that superheroes have? Well, some of them do, but a lot of them don't. Let's talk about what you can do to get enough exercise to be really pretty without knocking yourself out every day unless you want to. If you want to, more power to you, it will only help you be pretty and there's nothing wrong with that.

Can you get away with not doing any exercise at all? The truth is that you can sometimes get way with this if you are really young. If you are older than thirty though, you really need to do at least some exercise. It is recommended for younger pretty girls too.

So what do you really have to do? What you really have to do to stay pretty is just a little bit of exercise each day. I highly recommend some sort of yoga stretching when you get up in the morning to keep your limbs limber. As we age we start to set up like a gelatin and we lose that flexibility unless we exercise it daily. Yoga stretches do feel really good in the morning and can take less than five minutes. If you are nice and limber not only is it pretty, but you are less likely to hurt yourself doing everyday things.

I also recommend doing some kind of upper body strengthening in the morning. We tend to have lots of strength in our legs because we use them, and less in our arms because we tend to be lazy as a species unless we have a job loading or unloading boxes. If we have a job like that we are good to go and no other exercise is needed.

For the rest of us who need easy basic upper arm exercises, resistance bands are a good choice. You don't need a gym; just a twenty dollar set of resistance bands that you can hang over your door or work with isometrically. Check out the internet and Google for resistance band exercises. Just pick a couple of exercises that target where you think you need work and do maybe ten to twenty reps per day. That's all!

It takes less than five minutes. You can do a five minute workout if you do it every day and get results. Just get it over with in the morning and in a couple of weeks you will start to see muscle definition where you didn't have any before.

What else do you need for exercise? Aerobics. You need to get that blood pumping just a little for cardiovascular health and that rosy cheek factor. Pretty girls are strong and don't become winded doing simple tasks. They make everything look easy peasy.

What type of exercise should you do? Anything that counts. If you are spending an hour vacuuming, that counts as aerobic exercise. If you take a half hour walk over lunch, that counts as exercise. If you golf or play tennis, this counts. If you go to a theme park and walk around, that counts. Just do anything you can to keep your blood moving and it counts! Try to go for a half hour of some kind of movement every day.

If you are lucky enough to find some exercise classes that really make you happy then go for that. Some people like Zumba or Bollywood style dancing. Maybe you prefer ballet or tap. Some places even offer Cirque du Soleil style acrobatics with trapezes, hoops, or aerial fabrics hanging from the ceilings. If you like the classes you could go once or twice a week, and then just take walks or switch it up on the other days. No need to go every day unless you really want to. It is not necessary to do these classes, you can absolutely do your exercises at home, but it will up your fitness factor even more if you choose to go for it. Fit equals pretty!

7

CLOTHING

STYLE

Clothing is sometimes synonymous with style; at least we'd like it to be. Style is something that every pretty girl has. For some it is intuitive, for others it takes careful study. There are three basic styles that pretty girls tend to lean towards. These styles are classic, girly, or elegant. If you don't like these styles can you still be pretty? Of course. But choosing one of these styles and incorporating them into a style you already like will make being pretty easier.

Famous pretty girls with a classic style include Natalie Portman, Kate Middleton, Jennifer Aniston, and Kate Winslet. Classic style is all about moderation. It is about simple lines and classic colors. You won't find any eighties neon in these wardrobes. These girls tend not to follow the trends unless a trend becomes a classic, and this takes time. They like to wear well-cut clothing that flatters the lines of their natural shapes, and they like to wear natural fabrics. There is nothing frilly or frivolous about the classic style.

Famous pretty girls who dress in the girly style include Keira Knightley, Amanda Seyfried, Katy Perry, and Zooey Deschanel. These girls like to be feminine! You won't find them in something masculine or fashions that they consider to be drab; those styles are boring to them. They like to play with fun bright colors and feminine styles. They are especially fond of dresses, and like to wear pastels here and there. They want everyone to know that they are a girl and they aren't afraid to show it. Twirly dresses with full skirts are popular with this crowd.

Famous pretty girls who use the elegant style include Angelina Jolie, Cate Blanchett, Sofia Vergara, and Scarlett Johansson. These girls are kind of a hybrid mix between girly and classic. They chose beautiful, elegant clothing with a feminine flair. They look clean and graceful, and invest in quality clothing. They wear colors that do not overly contrast with their own coloring. Gently muted, and refined darker hues are the colors these girls tend to reach for.

Do you have to choose one of these styles to be a bona fide pretty girl? No, but it won't hurt you if you do. Once you choose a style, try to make all your future clothing purchases fall in line with the type of pretty girl you'd like to be. There are always crossovers of course. You can be classic and elegant and also throw in a touch of sophisticated. You can go with romantic or glamourous, which meshes well with the girly or elegant styles. You can use a bit of chic in your classic style, or add a touch of arty or bohemian to girly or classic.

The styles you want to use less of are punk, flamboyant, western, goth, or rocker. Can you infuse these styles into yours and still be pretty? Yes, but be careful not to overdo it. If you really love western, just use a touch in your clothing, like a western bracelet or belt buckle. Don't go with full out western gear unless you are going line dancing. You can creep into cartoon territory when using these styles exclusively, and your pretty won't be taken as earnestly.

The style I caution against most is the athletic style. Athletic style clothes are really only meant for the gym. There has been an infusion of lazy girls wearing these styles outside of the gym because the clothing is comfortable. The clothing manufacturers have sold them a bill of goods saying that it's okay to look like a sloth. But these clothes are never for pretty girls unless they are actually at the gym, running, or working out. Athletic clothes tend not to be as flattering as other styles, and they make it look like a lack of effort has been made. Sweatpants away from the gym say girls have given up on life, and don't care about their appearance. There is a big difference between looking like you didn't try too hard, and looking like you didn't try at all. If you see a pretty girl wearing these clothes it is because she is pretty despite the clothes and not because of them. Can you imagine how much prettier she would be if she just wore some pretty girl clothes?

Another lovely way to style yourself is to pick an influential fashion decade and take your cues from that. Some of the great decades for clothing were the thirties, forties, fifties and sixties. Look up these fashions and try to find examples of clothing in the girly, elegant, or classic styles and use them with a modern twist. Just a word of caution though, don't ever wear a style from a decade you can remember. This will age you faster than progeria. You will look like you got into a trend a long time ago, and never updated your look. If you are a fan of the eighties, and remember it, you can't wear that stuff and look pretty.

ACCENTUATE THE POSITIVE

It is imperative that you know your positive traits and that you exploit them to the best of your abilities. Pretty girls always accentuate the positive. They know what their most fabulous characteristics are and they put the focus on those things. Think you don't have any fabulous traits? Then look harder. You have them, I promise. Everyone has something that other people wish they had.

Maybe you are stick thin and clothes hang really well on you. Maybe you are sporting a nice rack. Maybe your hair is like spun gold or rich silk. Maybe you have a tiny waist. Maybe your skin is really smooth and pretty, your teeth are white and straight, or you have a mega-watt smile. Maybe you have deep set eyes or killer lashes. Maybe your legs are long and toned. Find whatever it is about yourself that totally rocks and draw attention to that trait.

No matter how heavy you think you are, never wear a sack or a mumu. This just makes you look heavier! And it doesn't accentuate a nice figure if you are not heavy. Don't do it. If you have a dress like this that you love and won't part with, get it tailored. A great way to have your clothes look fabulous on you is to have a tailor on hand. Once you find an affordable tailor who you can trust, put them on speed dial! Here is your tailor's job: to make those clothes that only sort of or mostly fit you into the clothing of your dreams.

The tailor's work is to help you accentuate the positive and make the clothes hang on you like they were made for you, and essentially they are being fashioned for you. I can't even tell you what a huge difference a good tailor makes. They can bring that waist in right at your slimmest spot to make you look more slender. They can loosen the bust so that the fabric falls in a flattering way. They can make clothing the perfect length for you.

The most flattering length for a dress is just below the knee. You ideally want it to touch just where your calf begins to take on fullness just below your knee. This makes your legs look shapely and your torso appear to be just the right height and ratio.

One of the styles of dresses that seems to work consistently on a lot of girls is the fit and flare style. These dresses are tight around the bust and looser around the waist. If you have a nice bust the focus will be on that. Maybe your waist is thicker than you'd like it to be. The flare will totally hide that, while making you appear more feminine. By the same token if you are stick thin all over, this style will still look nice on you, confirming that your bust is still bigger than your waist, no matter how small the girls may be. Of course I would recommend using a push-up bra to get the most you can out of this style, but it will still look lovely if you use it to go slightly boyish, yet still feminine.

Here's another rule of thumb: Always wear a tight top with a flowy bottom, or a tight bottom with a flowy top. You can sometimes get away with a form fitting top and tight bottoms if you are going to a concert or dinner, but never ever wear flowy and flowy together. This flowy and flowy will make you look like you are wearing a sack (not flattering on anyone) and like you have no idea what you are doing fashion-wise. But a pair of tight jeans with a flowy top is beautiful and modern. A flowy skirt with a form fitting top will accentuate your bust and downplay generous hips. Just keep this fashion rule in mind.

For swimwear I highly recommend ruching. It hides all the imperfections and makes you look really hot. Try to avoid two pieces unless you can really rock them. The most flattering two piece styles according to Cindy Crawford are the triangle adjustable tops with the adjustable tie bottoms. Anyone who can rock a bikini can rock this style.

With one piece swimwear I also recommend shapewear. Walmart has a great and affordable line called Suddenly Slim that is shapewear and swimwear in one. You'll be amazed how you look in these styles. There are other more expensive designers like Jantzen that also make swim shapewear. Get a push-up bathing suit too if you can find one. A bigger bust will always make your waist look smaller.

ACCESSORIES

A cornerstone of any pretty girl wardrobe includes accessories. Learning how to accessorize can make the difference between pretty and blah or mad hatter.

One of the biggest mistakes the girls make when accessorizing is overdoing it with the accoutrements. Choose one or two pieces of flair, and that's it! Wear a necklace and a bracelet or a necklace and earrings, but don't wear all three. Wear a scarf and a brooch instead of jewelry, but don't wear those two things with jewelry. Wear two necklaces together for a funky vibe, but leave the rest of the jewelry off. Or just wear the necklace by itself.

Hats count as accessories except for winter hats so keep that in mind. A large flower or a piece of hair jewelry in your tresses will count as an accessory as well.

A sweater or a blazer can be considered an accessory if it is interesting enough. If you have a blue velvet blazer or a fifties sweater with flowers sewn on it, this can be considered an accessory; it doesn't just have to be jewelry. Think outside the box. Again, you want it to look like you tried, but not too hard. You care about your appearance, but you don't want it to look as though you were so insecure about your pretty that you threw on everything in your closet.

The same rule that applies to accessories also applies to color, only with a stricter limitation. If you are going to wear a bright color, wear only one thing. Wear a bright top with neutral-colored pants. Wear a brightly patterned skirt with a black or gray top. Better yet, just wear a pop of color on your otherwise neutral palette. Try a bright blue or red fabric rose pinned to your sweater, or a brightly colored belt or necklace with your more muted hues. A muted pink or blue can count as a neutral. Just try to avoid having too many brights together.

For shoes, try to keep them neutral if you are rocking a brightly-colored pretty dress or a stunning sweater. Remember, only one or two pieces of flair. Black shoes especially, and whites and nudes, look best for all fashions. If you have a pair of really wild shoes that you love and want to wear, make sure the rest of your outfit is dark, neutral, or black to show off those stunning pumps.

I have a pair of Zombie Stompers from Iron Fist that I love. They are bright yellow with eyeballs and teeth on them. Those shoes are awesome, and totally psychobilly. The only thing I can really wear them with though is a black dress, or jeans and a black top. Anything else steals attention from their awesomeness. But when I do wear them with that black dress, the compliments roll in.

Scarves are one of the easiest and most sophisticated accessories that exist. These things are like magic for dressing up your wardrobe. If you are wearing a neutral tee and jeans and you throw on a fabulous scarf, suddenly you have transformed into a fashionista! You totally look like you know what you are doing when you don one of these things, especially if you are following the rule about only one or two pieces of flair. Just throw on the scarf if that's all you have time for and you are rocking it!

8

FASHION MISTAKES

SABOTAGE

Fashion mistakes are things that sabotage or take away from pretty. The thing about these mistakes, though, are that they are totally preventable! In this chapter we will discuss ten common fashion mistakes and how to prevent them. Sometimes being pretty isn't just about what you do; it's about what you don't do. Just don't block the light and let the pretty shine through.

LEGGINGS

Here's the thing about leggings. Leggings are not pants! This is the number one fashion mistake I see girls making. Leggings look ridiculous when worn without something covering them. They look as if a girl started to get dressed and then decided not to bother, or simply forgot to put on a skirt over it.

Girls make the mistake of thinking it's fine to do this because they see the models online posing in the advertised leggings with nothing covering them to show them off, but the models online also model bras without a shirt, and the bras are not meant to be worn without one.

Leggings with a short mini skirt are fine. Leggings with a tunic or a long enough top to cover your bum are fine too. Leggings worn as pants look ridiculous. No fashionista worth her salt would be caught half-dressed, and you shouldn't either!

If you really love the feel of leggings by themselves, the fashion industry has created a solution for this: they are called jeggings, and they are meant to be worn as pants. They are a legging-jeans hybrid that you may already have in your closet. They are almost every bit as comfortable as a legging.

SHORTS

Shorts should almost never be worn. They look so

terrible that the European Fashion Union has banned them.   Okay, this isn't exactly true, but people don't wear them over there in our fashion-forward sister countries. The only country shorts are really worn in is the United States, and other countries make fun of us to no end for this.

There is one exception to this rule. If you look like you are under 30 you can wear jean shorts, but no other kind if you want to look like a pretty girl. If look over 30, just give them up completely and you'll be doing yourself a huge favor.   Most shorts are not fashionable; they just look frumpy. And if you are older and wearing them you will just look like you are trying to recapture your youth, which never works, it just looks sad.

Of course if you are playing a sport such as volleyball where shorts are de rigueur, then you can use them where appropriate.

BRAS AND UNDERWEAR

There are only two colors of underwear you need in

your closet. Those colors are nude and black. Why did I not list white? Because it's another top ten fashion mistake. I'm not sure where women got the idea that they should wear white underwear and bras under white shirts, but it is woefully untrue. The only color that should be worn under white is nude. It's the only color that won't show.

Look around the next time you go out. When you see girls wearing white shirts or dresses, you will immediately be able to tell if they are wearing white underwear, and they are a walking fashion ticket or not. I see it all the time.

Another mistake women often make is letting their bra straps show. This looks ridiculous if not done properly. The absolute worst way you can do this is to wear thin nude adjustable bra straps that show. If you are going to make this fashion mistake by wearing a regular bra that shows, at least make it look deliberate by wearing a bold color like red or purple. It makes no sense to let a nude bra show; they are nude because they are not meant to be seen.

The proper way to wear the visible bra strap trend

is to get a bralette with thicker straps; one that looks like it might or might not actually be a bra, but could be a top underneath your shirt. The lacy ones are especially good for this. Aerie has a great selection of showable bralettes, particularly the racerback ones. If you put those tiny adjustable straps on display it just looks like your underwear is showing. It looks unintentional and like you don't know what you are doing fashion-wise. Fashion should always look intentional.

PANTY LINES

Don't let them show. Panty lines are not meant to be seen. This is another thing that will have people noticing the fashion mistake on your bum instead of looking at your pretty face or figure.

There are pantyline-free panties advertised as such that are pretty good at not showing under your clothing, so try to get some of those if you don't have them already. Always check your backside before you leave the house.

Thong underwear is another option if it's right for you, but please don't let those show on the upper or waist side of your garments either. People will just be staring at your underwear, and not at your pretty.

Commando's patches are another great option. These are disposable cotton patches that you stick right into the crotch of your pants. You will never have panty lines again if you wear these so if anyone looks at your bum, it's because your bum looks nice, not because there's a fashion mistake on it.

TAGS

Many ladies out there do not bother to cut the tags out of their shirts. This is why companies like American Eagle and Hollister have started printing the tags on the back of the shirts, so people who wear their clothing don't go around looking like idiots. Harsh, but true.

If you do not buy clothing from companies that print the tag info on the inside of the shirt itself, please cut out the tag. Those little things just stick out and they attract attention. They make it look as though you are the absent-minded professor; not all together there, and not polished.

If, for whatever reason, you refuse to cut the tags, just make sure you check for their visibility before you leave the house. I always see people pointing at those on other people. They definitely take away from pretty.

FANNY PACKS

These little horrors were invented in the 1980's. Not to date myself, but even then I recognized them for the terrors that they truly were. Oh sure, it's great to be hands-free, if you don't mind looking really dreadful and slovenly. These things are ugly and terrible. You should never, ever wear a fanny pack if you want to be really pretty.

They stick out as an extension of your waist and they make it look like you have an extra deposit of fat just sitting on your tummy. Nobody needs that. Not even skinny minnies. Also they look really utilitarian.

Like you don't care what you look like because you are all about practical. It's fine to be practical, but don't sacrifice pretty for it! There are other ways, my beauty.

If you need to be hands-free, wear a cross body bag, or even a little backpack if you can find a cute one that's fashionable. If you are going hiking you can wear an honest to goodness JanSport backpack and still be pretty, but do not wear a fanny pack. Or here's another option: put all your essentials in your pockets. Scale down, carry less, it's prettier!!

But I'm a dress kind of girl, you say? There are dresses with pockets. I recommend the site eShakti where they will customize their dresses to fit you and you will receive them in only a week or two. These dresses come pre-tailored to your measurements for a very small fee, and they almost always have nice pockets!

ELASTIC WAISTBANDS AND SWEATS

Elastic waistbands are great for the manufacturers

because they can produce less sizes that will fit more people. They are good for consumers too, because it is easier for you to find a better fit. However, they are not good for pretty or for fashion. These little babies that show up in the stores (and maybe even in your wardrobe) are not meant to be seen. Not at all.

If you find a skirt you like with an elastic waistband, make sure you wear a fitted shirt that goes over it so it does not show. You can also wear a belt. There is a danger in this though because belts tend to slip and expose the elastic from time to time so if you choose to remedy the situation with this option, make sure your belt doesn't slip. It looks really cheap when they do.

Now for sweats. I've said this in other ways but it bears repeating: do not wear sweats outside of a workout situation. It's just fine for working out because it's the right situation for sweats. But you wouldn't wear a golf shirt and skort to a wedding. It might look hot on the golf course, but you wouldn't look pretty in that at the nuptials, right? Part of being pretty is wearing exactly the right thing for the occasion. It has to look like you effortlessly know what you are doing.

I realize that many Americans are getting lazy and just wearing what is comfortable, but don't be that lazy. Find a better way. I have always said you don't have to sacrifice comfort for pretty. You can wear something soft that fits you awesomely, and is super relaxed, and still be pretty.

FREE TEES

That event that you went to sure was fun, wasn't it? They even gave to a free t-shirt so you could remember the occasion. You are tempted to wear it because it shows everyone that you went to this event and you're cool, right? Well, don't ever wear them. There are a couple of reasons why.

The first reason is because they are usually one cut fits all, men and women (even if they say they have women's sizes) and the cut is terrible. It will look like a sack on you, it will not flatter your curves or your pretty figure. It will just make you look dumpy.

The second reason is that it is free advertising for the company. That's why they gave it to you in the first place. I don't know about you, but if I'm going to be advertising for someone, I'm going to be getting paid for it. If they want me to wear their ill-fitting tee-shirt, they need to fork over some compensation.

If you really want to remember the occasion, choose some other object that is reminiscent of the event. Maybe an electronic toy, or a bracelet. If you went to Disney, wear a tee-shirt that has subtle mickey ears or a silhouette on it, not one that says Disney all over it.

Let's say you really like the design of your free tee and you don't mind advertising for free. The cut is still going to be crappy unless you went to a fashion show. Cut the logo part of the tee out and sew it (or have it sewn) into you own great fitting tee, or onto the back of a moto jacket. That will make you pretty and cool, and you'll stand out from the crowd.

TOO MUCH CLEAVAGE

Ladies, it's wonderful if you have awesome cans. I understand the desire to show them off, but you have to leave a little something to the imagination to be really pretty. Unless you are auditioning for a Penthouse centerfold, you don't want to have your knockers all out on display.

Yes, nice breasts are awesome, but they do fall under the category of being distracting and taking away from pretty. When you have those on parade, everyone will be looking at them and only them. They won't notice if you're really pretty, because they won't be able to take their eyes off of your chest.

It's fine to show a little cleavage. Just make sure it doesn't extend to your belly button. If you have a nice figure and you are dressing appropriately, people will notice your face and also your figure. Wear a form fitting top, for instance, if you'd like to show your ladies off. It can be more alluring to show a little less skin because people may wonder what you've got hiding underneath.

FLIP FLOPS

Flip flops are a fashion disease everywhere, especially in the summer. They are particularly troubling year-round in places like Florida. People think that because it's hot outside, it's okay to wear flip flops all the time. Or because there's a beach nearby, it's okay to wear them 24/7. Now I am not talking about nice sandals that happen to have a thong toe; I am talking about the cheap plastic things you wear to the beach.

It's not okay to wear these outside of the beach or pool – not if you want to be really pretty. They're so cheap looking that I would even caution you not to wear them to the beach. I don't, but it's okay if you really like them for that. Again, you want the outfit to be appropriate for the occasion.

Really pretty girls wear real shoes. In the summer they wear comfortable sandals that look like sandals. They can be easy slip-on and have a thong toe, but they have to have a nice thick sole, or some pretty flowers on them that aren't made of plastic, or maybe a metal detail that spiffs them up.   Again, there are ways to be comfortable and pretty too!

9

CLASS

YOU CAN HAVE CLASS

To be really pretty, you've got to have class. You may believe that class is one of those things that you just have or you don't. This is true in some cases. However, class can be cultivated. If you don't already have all the down low on how to have it, here are some tips.

STAY CALM

Pretty girls don't go around creating mayhem like crazy maniacs. Pretty girls have sophistication and they are calm under pressure. Whatever happens to you in your daily life, there is no good to be had from flying off the handle or freaking out. Even (and especially) in life threatening emergencies, it is best to have a calm demeanor.

Classic screen beauties like Elizabeth Taylor and Katherine Hepburn always found a way to handle a tricky situation in a composed manner. Did this detract from their allure because they weren't yelling and screaming or drawing attention to themselves? Of course it didn't. It made them seem capable, and even more attractive, especially to their male co-stars who were often astonished at the mettle that made up these women.

So let's say that life has decided, as it sometimes does, to take a swing at you. Everything was going your way and then wham, you get hit with something unexpected that really causes your blood to boil, or worse, causes you to panic. What can you do to not spoil your clothing, your make-up, or your radiant expression? Take a deep breath.

This may be the same advice that you've heard over and over again. It's so trite that you may no longer even consider it as an option. But the advice is commonplace because it works. Taking a breath allows oxygen to permeate your brain, which will allow you to think better and more clearly. It also gives you something to do while you are considering how to react to a certain situation. There is a pause between event and reaction. This will give you time to create a strategy for dealing attractively and effectively with your problem.

Following your breath, think about what the next step is to solving the problem. Ask yourself what is the very next logical thing you can do that is helpful. Then do that thing even if it is only a little thing. More solutions will come into your head after you take that first little step. It is almost never helpful to scream unless you are being attacked in a public place and someone might be able to come to your assistance. Usually screaming just mucks things up and doesn't do anything to solve the difficulty.

Even if you don't know what to do, just do the first thing you can think of that doesn't make the situation worse. People around you will admire your calm response, and you will look more beautiful because of it. And because you are calm, people may be more willing to lend their assistance if you should need it. Pretty girls are no longer damsels in distress; pretty girls are capable and wise.

CONSIDER BEFORE ACTING

This advice goes hand in hand with the last tenet. But "consider before acting" addresses how to not put your foot in your mouth or act rashly. Feet in mouths are not attractive. Rash responses are also not always pretty.

I know it may seem like you have to be really lively and keep the conversation going quickly in order to be pretty. This can sometimes work if you are really on top of your game, but it cannot be sustained, and there is a surer footed way.

Think before you act. You can be slow and thoughtful in your responses. Beauty queens don't have to snap to attention and immediately reply or act to a question or command. Pretty girls can look calm; they can slowly and gracefully mull it over before anything comes out of their fetching mouths. You will find that people will wait for you.

If you give a considered reply, you will look smarter. If you don't look rushed, people will believe that because you take your time, you are worth listening to. Society has taught women to be people-pleasers, so we will often come up with quick answers and responses to others so as to be polite and not keep people waiting.

But you are a pretty girl. You are worth more than that. You can show people your worth by waiting until you have something clever or useful to say. People will appreciate you more for your brain, which will in turn make your outer form more beautiful. Girls who take their time show others that they are pretty, and worthwhile.

If you are unsure that you should say or do something, first consider the consequences. If you are going to say something unkind to someone, will it really make you feel better? Or will you be regretting it later? Sometimes if something needs to be said, it needs to be said. But hold on, until you are sure. Maybe there is a kinder way to say it that will make you look more attractive. The metaphorically bigger person will always seem better looking.

BE GENEROUS

Pretty girls are generous girls. They are generous with their spirit, and their kindness. Stingy people just aren't that attractive.

Go the extra mile, especially if it doesn't cost you much. For instance, be the pretty girl that always sends out Christmas cards. It is a little thing, but seems very generous to your friends and family.

Be the girl who always says please and thank you. Manners are generous and attractive. People appreciate them because it shows others that they are worthy of respect, and that they have value. This elevates you in their eyes, and makes you look pretty to them.

Be generous with your time. I don't mean that you have to say yes to every bake sale. If you love bake sales, then feel free! But be generous to people when you are with them in the time that you have together.

When people are talking to you, be generous with

your attention. Pay full consideration to them. Act like they are the only person in the room when you are speaking with them. Look them in the eye. Girls who do this are a dying breed, and doing this just ups the beauty factor for them.

Things you can do to be generous are little things. You can offer people a glass of water. You can buy people small gifts (like a bookmark if they are a reader) when you see something that makes you think of them. You can sit down with someone and lend them your ears if you get the impression that they need to talk.

The most generous thing you can do for people that will probably do the most for both of you and for your prettiness, is to give them your smile. I can't even tell you how many people compliment me on my smile on the days that I use it. A smile is a huge gift to other people – it tells them that they are okay, and that everything else is going to be okay, even if it seems like it's not. Smiles are super inexpensive and they offer a fantastic return on investment.

GIVE TIPS

Tipping makes you look generous and beautiful. Tipping is not about the person being tipped. Tipping is about the person doing the tipping. If you remember Steve Martin in *My Blue Heaven*, he always said, "I tip everybody!" And everyone loved him. This generous attitude made him more attractive, did it not?

Yes, sometimes it is a pain to always have cash on hand for tipping. But it is a part of society. If you do not tip you are considered classless and stingy. No one wants to be thought of a as miser. Misers are not attractive, are they? They just sit on their little pile of money with their mouths in a twisted sneer.

Class includes generosity. When you are generous, you are open, and people like you. It is true that you can be beautiful and hated, but it is a lot tougher to keep that up than if you are beautiful and generous. People will overlook any flaws you may believe you have if you are a generous person.

I remember before I was married when I used to go on dates, and I would always check to see how much my date tipped the waiter. That would tell me a lot about the guy I was dating, and might determine whether a second date or even a goodnight kiss was on the table.

One time I was so embarrassed by my date's tip that I made an excuse and went back to add more money to the check. You can guess whether that guy got a kiss or a second date. Yes, a man's attractiveness factor is affected by this too. Men automatically seemed more handsome to me if they were good tippers. I appreciated their willingness to share with others.

So here's the general rule: you tip anyone who touches your things. It doesn't have to be a lot, but it has to be something. People are watching you and looking at you and judging your attractiveness. Show them you are beautiful! In restaurants, tip at least twenty percent – at least twenty-five percent if they are awesome or they give you free stuff. If anyone touches your luggage, tip one dollar per bag at least. If you stay in a hotel, leave two to five dollars for the maids who will clean your room.

These tips will not make or break your bank, but

the people who work for these tips will be grateful. Other people always notice whether people tip or not, so make sure you are well-reflected; it is classy to tip properly!

REPLY

It is also classy to reply. People don't like to be ignored, and they like to think they are important to you. If you do not reply to their phone call or email or text, they might start to think of you as bitchy and your attractive factor will decrease in their eyes.

This does not mean that you have to reply immediately to every summons, but at least try to get back to people within twenty four hours. If you do not have time for a phone call, just send them a text or an email and let them know that you will get back to them in more depth as soon as you have time.

Girls who are so self-absorbed that they cannot be bothered to respond to others are not the girls who win the contest for prom queen. The prom queens are the ones who are open-hearted and generous to others, and make every person feel that they are important.

Why would you want to make anyone else feel "less than" anyway? You probably know what that's like, and if you don't you are lucky, but perhaps you can imagine. People who lift others up are the pretty people in our society. They are the ones that people will talk about with respect and admiration.

Pretty girls are the ones who send Christmas Cards and Thank-You Notes and get back to their friends as soon as they possibly can, letting their friends know that they are important. When you make someone feel important, you will become more beautiful to them.

So, if someone takes the time to contact you, just take a second to contact them back. Especially if they have done something to help you! Not only does this increase the likeliness that they will help you again, but it makes you look great.

Again, just a word or a text is all it takes to let someone know that they are important. That's all anyone ever really wants – to seem important to others.

When you exhibit this behavior, it sets you apart as being super classy, and it will help you seem just as pretty on the inside as you are by this time on the outside. This will increase your pretty factor by at least fifty percent.

10

ATTITUDE

THE RIGHT ATTITUDE

Of course pretty is about grooming and clothing and make-up and hair. But what else is pretty about? Well, by and large, pretty is very much about attitude. This is good news, because even if you don't have the perfect figure, or the perfect clothes and hair, you can still pull off pretty with the right attitude. This chapter will tell you how.

UNIQUENESS

The thing about pretty is that it has to be unique in some way to be really outstanding. You can be a Barbie doll, and Barbies are really pretty. But you know who's prettier than a Barbie doll? Angelina Jolie. That girl is unique! I'll use her for this example. Physically, her lips are a little too wide, and her head is a little too big for her body, but she's gorgeous.

What else makes her pretty? Her attitude. She is a really different girl. She kissed her brother on the mouth at the academy awards, she flies airplanes, and she once wore a vial of her husband's blood around her neck. She has insane tattoos galore. Are all of these things awesome? No, undoubtedly some are bizarre. But when you add it all up, it equals her uniqueness, which makes her crazy gorgeous.

The thing about pretty girls is that they are not afraid to be themselves. They are not afraid to show their true colors even if it defies convention. Do I suggest that you do these strange Angelina Jolie things? No. I am suggesting that you do your own wild things that show the world that you are beautiful. Yes, Angelina knows how to put herself together and that helps a ton. But what makes her even prettier? Her strangeness. The strangeness that comes straight from her soul. I know you have that too.

Just to be clear, I am not suggesting that you break the law. Keep it legal; mug shots are not pretty. And don't go too crazy with it. Pretty girls are off-kilter just enough to make them edgy; not enough to send them to the nut house. If you feel like streaking down the street in nothing but your birthday suit, maybe try doing it in your underwear on a snowy day instead. At least you won't get arrested.

Maybe you have an unusual signature fragrance that you always wear. Maybe you like to express yourself with clothing. Perhaps there's a peculiar necklace that you bought in Peru that you like to model. Maybe you have a gap tooth or a crooked smile. Whatever it is that makes you off-kilter will also make you more beautiful! Find the unusual or bizarre in you and express it just a little bit.

POISE AND POSTURE

Pretty girls stand up straight. If you stand up straight it automatically looks like you are full of confidence, and this comes off as very pretty. Yes, Angelina is weird and wacky, but do you ever see her slouch? Rarely. It is also important to sit up straight as often as you can. If you didn't go to a boarding school or have a modeling agency mother then this is tough! But it is necessary.

The slouching habit is a ruinous one. Not only does it scream unprofessional and shrinking violet, but it can be harmful to your health! This posture will prey on your muscles and spinal cord and cause you back problems when you get older. When you stay in that position all the time, Mother Nature will accept it and will conspire to keep you that way.

Do you really want to be a hunched-over old lady? I feel so bad for these people when I see them. Also, when I see younger girls with a super slump, I know it's only going to get worse when they get older, and a slump like that isn't pretty! Start now. The sooner you make it a habit in your life, the easier it will become!

Holding yourself up high gives you poise. Poise is defined as graceful, elegant, and balanced. Poise is super pretty. Ballerinas have poise! So keep your back straight and keep your actions deliberate. Part of poise is being a little bit methodical. If you are deliberate instead of haphazard, you will appear more confident.

Be balanced and graceful. If you practice grace

you can achieve it. If you are not sure how to be graceful, study women who you think have poise, and then emulate them. You will automatically start to practice elegance when you straighten out that back. It gives you a feeling of confidence that, if you don't at first feel, you will start to relax into.

So place those shoulder blades back and down, and keep your head up and your chin slightly back. It might feel a little awkward at first if you are not used to having good posture. But if you can ease into it, it will start to feel natural. If you are not used to this, to begin with you may feel as if others think you are trying to be superior by having such good posture (most people don't), but if it becomes a part of you, no one will question it.

ACCEPTING HELP

Of course pretty girls are self-sufficient, but sometimes others want to help, especially if you are pretty, so let them! I know that often it is men who will want to help pretty girls by opening doors for them, or lifting luggage for them on an airplane, and I also know that some girls are insistent on being feminist and showing the world that they can cope with life without the aid of anyone else.

But if you accept help when it is offered, you will seem prettier. People have to go out of their way to offer to help someone else. It is not always an easy thing to do. So if you reject their offer of help, you may cause them to feel stupid and useless. They are helping you because it makes them feel good, particularly if you are pretty.

You don't want to make others feel like they went out of their way to be kind and were rejected. You want them to feel good that they offered you help. If you reward them with a kind smile, that is often all the validation they need. They may go back into their day with a proverbial skip in their step because they helped someone pretty.

You will definitely seem prettier if you accept their help rather than reject it. If you don't act like a ninny, everyone will know that you can lift your own bag if that is important to you. Of course the exception to accepting help is this: don't accept it from people who don't seem right to you, always trust your gut.

However, if you do actually need help, don't be afraid to look around and see if anyone is paying attention. Look politely and see if there is an offer. If not, then try it yourself, and if you can't seem to lift that bag, then politely ask someone who looks strong to help you with it. That said, don't carry on more than you can lift. Flight attendants do not get paid to lift luggage.

If you start to be prettier you will notice more people attempting to help you. You should try to get comfortable with this. People doing things like opening doors for you will become the new norm. Again, everyone wants to be a part of a pretty person's orbit, so if you can, let them.

SMILE AND LAUGH

Smiling does wonders for your face. It shows people that you are friendly, and if you are not super young, it can take years off of your appearance. Pretty girls, when they are not doing a beauty mug for the camera, smile a lot. I think that many of them have come to see this as necessary.

They feel that if they don't smile, then people will think that they are stuck up, just because they are pretty. They want to re-assure everyone that this is not the case, and that that they treat all individuals equally and never act superior. Yes, there are a few pretty girls out there with a perpetual pout, but their beauty won't last. It's true what your mother said, "Your face will freeze that way!"

Not literally this second, but give it time. Ten to fifteen years of frowning will start to put those frowny lines on your face and it will eventually be frozen that way. If your face is going to have lines on it, they need to be the happy lines that keep you pretty, so try to smile as much as you can. Besides, studies have shown that the more you smile, the happier you will be.

Yes, you can use botox to rid yourself of those lines, but who wants to rely on such a heavy toxin all the time? Get Botox or surgery if it suits you, or if it's too late to erase years of frowning, but I would prefer to use those things as a last resort. Overdone, you face can freeze in a neutral expression and you won't have that pretty smile.

I once worked with a girl who had Botox done and she could only smile with half of her face. She didn't look nearly as pretty as the much older lady (with gray hair!) I worked with who was super kind and generous with her smiles.

Also, people usually look the most beautiful when they laugh! People love to see other people laugh. The resonant sound combined with the extravagant smile just makes people tingle with happiness. If you are one of those people that spreads that happiness around, then people will find you attractive. People love to be laughed at when they tell a joke or try to be funny. Try to help them dole out the happiness if you can.

ACT AS IF

Probably the single most important thing you can do

for your prettiness is to act as if you were pretty! If you act like you are pretty then people will pick up on that. If they don't think you are pretty at first, they will wonder why you are acting pretty. Since you are acting that way they may start to think they pegged you wrong, and that you actually are pretty. Then, they will also start to think of you as pretty since you so clearly see yourself that way.

I always think of the show Drop Dead Diva. In it, a really pretty girl who is a model dies and then goes to heaven. When she's at the computer desk and they are figuring out where to put her, she presses the return key on the keyboard. Then she gets jettisoned back into the world into the body of a plus-sized lawyer who has just died. She awakens in the substantial lawyer's body.

Is this overweight lawyer pretty at first blush? Decidedly not, especially if you compare her to the stick-thin model she used to be. But in the show she has to cope with the fact that she's been given a body that isn't model material. However, this girl is so used to acting like she is pretty, that she continues to do this. She carries herself like she is pretty, she dresses like she is pretty, and she flirts like she is pretty. She doesn't let her size stop her from acting pretty.

And you know what? We buy it! We buy every sexy twirl, every lingering look, and every knowing hair flip. If she's ignoring that fact that she isn't as pretty as she used to be, then we can too! It's all about attitude! She keeps up with fashion and she loves her glamorous celebrities. Like other pretty girls, instead of being jealous of beautiful superstars, she appreciates them, and she emulates them.

So do all the things that pretty girls do, and you too will be pretty. Even if you don't believe it as first, just act the part. I promise you that when you act as if you are pretty, people will start to treat you like you are. Once they start to treat you that way, you will relax into the role. It will become second nature, and you will be a bona fide pretty girl!

ABOUT THE AUTHOR

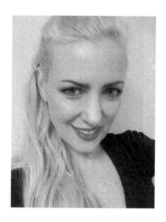

Bronwen Skye has starred in commercials, music videos, and made for cable television movies. She has appeared in Playboy magazine twice. She earned her fine arts degree in Theater from Marymount Manhattan College in New York City. She is the author and contributing author of several books, including fiction, nonfiction, and satiric poetry.

True to having broadened her horizons at an early age by spending some of her developmental childhood years in Africa, she is a professional traveler, and vegan food connoisseur. Following a move to Southern California, she wrote and hosted a radio show called Insight on AM 1460, and wrote an Op-Ed piece for the Santa Monica Outlook.

When she's not traveling around the country, she spends her time reading and writing fantasy horror young adult fiction, and practicing circus style acrobatics. A fanatic for all things Disney, she now lives in the Sunshine State with her 4 rescued felines and 1 rescued husband.

If you liked this book, we'd love to have your review on Amazon! If you didn't, please contact us at prettygirl@bronwenskye.com and let us know what we can do to make the next book better!!

If you are interested in finding out more about Bronwen Skye and to find out how to get the next book for free, just go to http://bkrepublic.wix.com/pretty.

Printed in Great Britain
by Amazon